THE BEGINNING OF MY IMMORTAL LIFE AND ETERNITY

Serge Dobrow

Copyright Page.

Dedication Page:

This work is dedicated to my lovely son who left us before time.

Contents

Foreword

About twenty-five years ago I worked with PhD Mr. Allen Omton in military lab that researched the possibility of remote communication between people in extreme situations, when other technical communication media is not functioning.

This secure lab worked under the high-level military supervision and was opened to unlimited access to any research teams, labs, colleges, and universities in country, and covered by unlimited budget.

All technical and experimental management in lab was conducted by Allen, and I was responsible for planning experiments with remote contacts.

The idea of remote contact was simple and require one or several people who need to pass and accept visual, textual, or emotional data with certain content.

The fact of possibility of such communication between people was well known before this lab had been created, and we started not from the zero level. Each lab worker had his own experience with remote communication and the main goal was in preparation the ordinary military staff for such unusual form of activity.

In the beginning, we demonstrated the ability of remote communication to the military management, and then lab had been created. We worked hardly for five years running hundreds of researches, tests, investigations, detail chemical and physical analyses provided by large number of scientific groups in different facilities.

The result was a bit unusual, and not as we suppose to receive. The success of data remote transaction was depended on the physical, emotional, and intellectual status of military staff participating in research. Some images that were slightly touched the mind of participants were transferred with high level of accuracy, and objects of meditations were not. Some fragments are transferred better than the main content, etc.

The satisfied level of remote communication has been reached only in special cases when participants were in special physical, emotional and intellectual stage. Allen call it "Zero Stage", when internal dialog is suppressed, and all energy centers are equally active.

Unfortunately for us, we can't require military staff to elevate they skills to the required level, and our lab was liquidated as failed to produce the achieved results.

Being depressed and disappointed, we united in our own lab under Allen's supervision to finish our research of the human's energy that changes the quality of remote communication.

Each of us had separate work where we were payed for living, and we worked in the lab as volunteers. Soon after, only three of us continue research, and the rest had left. We worked day and night by testing and monitoring different human's conditions when participants can clearly see or listen remotely. Once we got satisfied results, and assembled all researches in the report, Allen made an announcement that we made much more, than prove of remote communication. We found the way of tuning the human's energy and bringing it in resonance with other energies.

Each of us feels differently after experiments with remote communication. Our body was vibrating, the blood pressure was elevated, the mind was clear and intellectual activity was significantly jumped up.

We also accounted that our food choice was changed, chronical illnesses vanished, and the vision was improved. We become younger.

It was initially accepted as a joke, but by the close inspection, we found other changes in our body and mind.

It was a pandemic flu at the time when we work together, and all our coworkers become sick almost in the same time, except our team who didn't experience any symptoms of flu without taking flu shots that we simply forget to do being super overloaded by our work.

Our lab made shift in researches by experimenting with people who was sick, or aged. We had good relations with many labs and medical facilities, and it was no problem in getting medical support in these new researches. The result was very optimistic. People were changed to better under our training exercises.

Allen created the theory that he calls "Immortal Life Science". This theory confirms the human's ability to live immortal life without aging, pain, or illnesses.

He published all our researches in book [1] where all wisdom of our group where combined with his own ideas. He also asked us to publish our own books to promote the idea about immortality.

My immortal life started long time ago when the relevant terminology was unknown yet. We were on the top of our energy in conducting experiments with our body and mind by using different sources of modern and ancient techniques.

Year by year, these techniques and exercises were combined in the most effective methods improving the mind and body to get better results in our experiments. We were crazy in our dedication to get the result. Allen was the absolute fanatic and guru in our lab.

Later, we become separated after being married and live in different towns. I lost the communication with the rest of our team and write several letters to Allen. He answered with short and emotional sentences that we should let other people know about our research, and our goal is in making at least one more immortal person.

Allen and I could communicate with other immortals, but no one wish to write about they experience. Immortals believe that each person should find they own way to become immortal and should not to be "pushed" on this way until person is ready. One of immortals say that apple should be ready to be eaten before to be collected.

Allen Omton disagreed with this opinion, and decided to make our research available for public, expecting the great interest for such important subject.

He was wrong, and immortals were right. Allen's books were too complicated and published too early to be read and understood by ordinary public, and people simply rejected it as simply new religion, or philosophy.

He was somehow prepared to it and didn't regret about publishing. His next attempt was to make theory less complicated and affordable for anyone to understand.

My opinion on theory of immortal life is same as the opinion of the immortals, this theory is difficult to understand by public not because it is written by using complex language, but because the ordinary mind is not ready to accept the core idea of immortality and rejects it as "nonsense" or "fantasy".

What we can expect from people who knows from the childhood that all people are aging, become sick, and dying? All our society is built to accommodate this idea about mandatory death. I know that it is wrong, the immortals that I communicate, know that it is wrong, but we can't change mind of people in one attempt. All needs the time.

Immortals have this time, but what about mortal people? We feel so sad when people, who we know, died after straggling with illness, but we could help and save them. Allen always told us that it is our moral obligation to promote the knowledge about immortality to save at least more one soul.

When I talked to some immortals and asked them to come up publicly with they experience, I always received the cold face with refuse. "No one would be interested in my personal feelings or emotions" – was the answer. Some immortals afraid to become recognized by friends and coworkers who could negatively treat the immortality. Some my immortal friends could have the legal issues with the biological age that they hide in altered birth documents, etc.

I denied Allen's propositions to come up with my life experience to help other people since I didn't believe that anyone will be interested, and moreover, start they own immortal life. It was until I was witnessed of very sadden death of my son who could be alive now if I wouldn't keep my silence and be more persuasive. I overcome my wrong believes and decided to publish this book in memory of my son.

Here is my personal story that I would like to share with anyone who will be interested in eternal living with joy and happiness.

The Beginning

At the age of ten I had strange and remarkable night dream about some-one passed special knowledge in my memory. My parents told me many years later that I walked to the window with closed eyes, stayed several minutes, and then came back to my bed. I remember the face of person who talked to me, remember the image of space with colorful planets in it, and completely forgot the meaning of words that person was told. Only deep feeling of importance of the message was carved in my mind forever. Many times, I try to restore the meaning of what was said, but without success. Soon, I was consumed by my life, and gradually forgot this dream for a while.

At the age of sixteen I was presented by tiny book about Indian sacred system of elevation the body energy. It was a book about yoga translated on my language. I swallowed the book content during one night without any interruption and feel myself shivered like straitened by lighting.

Yoga becomes my everyday ritual that changed some my habits and believes. It was, probably, the moment, when my Immortality starts to form. I have no idea about eternal life, didn't read Bible, had very approximate knowledge about religions, and about zero knowledge about the personal energy.

My feelings of strange electrical current in my body cannot be classified at that time in any way, but excess of youth and desire.

The Europe at that time was consumed by social movements activated after the Second World War, and religions was not in favor, especially "wrong" religions was coming from other countries. Books about Buddhism, Samkhya, and Yoga, was missing in book stores, and a few of it were available in special libraries by limited access for special people. It was the time with no Internet available.

My hunger to knowledge about the most interesting books exceeds the limit and I wrote letters in other countries with attempt to get any books that could satisfy my hunger.

I received books from Hungary, Poland, Russia, Germany, and some other countries. My budget was not enough to pay for translation of these books, and I learned languages to translate it. At that time, I read Bible New Testament, and was amazed by it. Jesus becomes my guru icon. I can't find the Bible Old Testament, for some reasons, and once received it from England. My English was next to zero at that time, and I learned it to read. The same person sent me the report of Maharishi Mahesh Yogi that I translated with Old Testament during about a year or more. It was the time when I graduated the University and started my first work.

Bible Old Testament disappointed me a lot, since I expected something more than was in New Testament. Later I changed my mind by understanding that this historical book should be read first to prepare the reader's mind to accept Jesus teaching.

Jesus teaching and Indian philosophy somehow joined in my mind in the teaching about the real human being who should be free from impurities.

At that time social changes in my country becomes more loyal to religions and books come to me in the grate volume. I studied it, made notes, exercised, tried different system, approaches, and methods. My brain was working like crazy by processing tens of different approaches to human's perfection.

At that time I become consumed by the idea of Buddhism, and different types of yoga. It would be not necessarily to tell, how much time I spent in meditation, chanting mantras, performing kriyas, and physical exercises. I was pure vegan, and very slim, that makes my yoga easy to perform.

My personal energy was elevated up to the level when I could find other people who does the same as me, and I become a member of municipal club that united people interested in personal perfection.

We worked together, attending meetings and conferences, conducting the experiments, sharing the ideas, books, scrips, etc.

My knowledges jumped sharply, and I got the feedback from other enthusiastic people who walked in the same way as I did.

My everyday routine was substantially changed when I become married extraordinary young women that had her own vision on perfect life. My ego and absolute perfectionism was disassembled to the base that was crucial in my ascending to the idea about immortality.

The Idea about the Immortality

My visits and participation in club's life becomes rare, and I feel that I am losing the connection with my energy.

At that time, I received my Master of Computer Science degree, and my salary becomes a little higher, but steel was lower than married person can expect to live with dignity.

I opened small consulting company in the downtown, and use my knowledge to help people to resolve different problems in they life, including health, money, emotions, mental status, etc. It gives me better financial support and opens the broader access to club.

My friends didn't support my practice, deciding that I am losing my time by helping others and slowing down my own progress. I disagreed with this opinion being sure, that my personal energy benefits of my practice much more than solo exercises.

Once, my friend offered me the work with military research group that she supposed to manage. This group was created to investigate the possibility of remote contact between people without using any technical media. It was the fantastic opportunity to do the work that was my dream. The salary in military group was substantially higher than my occasional earning, and I agreed.

The research lab was formed by senior military command and included group lead who will report to military supervisor, scientific research lead, technical lead, couple people with the research experience, and several clerical workers.

At the time, when lab was almost formed, one of our club members Allen Omton defended his PhD sessions and becomes a lead of bilocation group. His expertise in research of paranormal effects was super ordinary. Allen was the star in our club due to his dedicated work and remarkable personality. He was tough to himself and club members, and newer allow to speculate in research transcriptions. He often says that he doesn't believe in anything, except he can personally tries, or touch. Allen was rock, who filters all "scientific researches" that failed to be explained by him and denied it as a fiction.

"We work to understand, and not to alter the facts" – he said. I loved and respected him very much and was shaking a bit when he reviewed my reports.

The rumors about extraordinary PhD Allen Omton came to attention of senior military staff and lab was suggested to be reordered in the way that Allen will invited to become the lead of lab. Allen publicly rejected this proposition as not aligned with his moral believes.

He was strong in his decision and newer came back to it until my friend asked him personally to accept this nomination instead of her. She was upset of changes in lab structure, since she was the one who brought the idea to the implementation, but the command from above was clear, that lab will be restructured or never created.

She was soft, nice, quiet and intelligent women, who created a lot activity around her, but trusted everyone and accepted any results without its scientifically strong analysis. Allen was not happy to commit such bad action as jump over someone's head, but she insisted on creation the lab, otherwise nothing will be created, and we could lose the opportunity.

Allen visited senior military meeting, and, finally, accepted the proposition. My friend was invited as the scientific researcher, but she refused and motivated it as unlikely military work environment for meditation. She was, probably, right, as we found out after five years of hard work in the lab.

Five years of crazy hard work with hundreds of experiments, dozens other scientific military and civil labs, conferences, meeting, tons of reports, are in front of us.

After five years we fail and win in the same time. We fail the main goal of lab, and military command withdraw the financing due to the lack of elaborated military procedure that can be used for military contingent to train them for remote communication.

The lab final report was reviewed by command, and came back with short notice, that fact of remote data transfer is proven to be existed in nature, and required special skills from participants that cannot be developed due to special military procedure. It constitutes our failure, and lab was dismissed.

By conducting multiple tests and researches we found that the successful data transfer was in the moment when personal energy is on rise. The participants, including us, and some military officers, reported about changes in physical, emotional, intellectual and social statuses. Many of them volunteered to participate in tests due to improving personal skills and better feelings.

These reports are not directly related to the goal of the lab but was registered by Allen with all his professional accuracy and advance vision. In some cases, we help military families in resolving difficulties in they life. Here my previous experience was in demand. Allen skeptically accepted my help to people, but not restricted it, since it helps in establishing better relations with military.

The lab closure did not surprise us since we understood the situations and was ready to retreat. Anyway, we were depressed by closure, and decided to continue our own investigations.

Allen offered all of us to stay and work without pay. All of us stay, but over the time we lost almost all staff, except three of us.

The lab was named by Allen as "long Life Style Company (LLSC)", and our goal was to find out the possible changes in ordinary mortal life to make it immortal.

We use the tons of publications collected in previous researches and created document with detail description of changes in human's body that, according to our understanding and experience, should change the life of ordinary person from mortal to immortal.

At that time our work was primarily with reports and papers, and we rarely conducted any experiments to try the immortal life on our own.

Time passed, and Allen was ready to publish our findings, but he was pending to make it available for public since we were not sure that all will work as planned.

He decides to keep the script on the shelf until we try the immortal life on our own life. We created the plan, our lab was dismissed, and Allen opened web site with LLSC publications to test the public interest to immortality.

After several years of testing the immortal life and periodic discussions results between three of us, Allen decided that it is a good time to go on public and print the book.

It was the time when the Internet becomes popular, and we discovered hundreds of Internet publications about the immortality, eternity, longevity, etc.

From the global search we found many social groups, where people decided to live and never die. Even before Internet search, we were familiar with immortals who communicate with us over the network. These people don't want to become publicly known and communicate only by the network. All our attempts to meet them personally was rejected, and the majority didn't support our attempts to make knowledge about immortal life known to the public.

Immortals believe, that secret knowledge, passed in wrong hands, can hurt people, disappoint them, and diminish the idea of eternal life. They believe that each human should grow the personal energy and become connected by network to other immortals to receive knowledge about immortality.

Allen and I discussed this condition and we didn't concluded the strategy. Allen believed that any one should know about the opportunity to live better life that is free of illnesses, safer, aging, and death. He told me, that, if one of thousand will save the life by changing it, then the goal will be reached, otherwise all our work is done for nothing, and it will become obsolete soon.

The decision was made by Anthony Ross, our third lab member, who stopped our disputes by declaring that ordinary person will accept or decline the idea about immortal life, depends on the personal energy. It means, that no risk is involved in publishing the theory of Immortality.

Anthony always bring the solid and right decision in our lab community. He worked a lot, but newer becomes tired. Anthony was very quiet, spent time in meditation, exercised yoga, and produced the best results in remote communication.

We were surprised that he supported the idea about going on public with the theory about immortality, since he always resists it. His point of view was the same as most immortals: keep secret knowledge available only for people who is ready to accept it.

Anthony said that anyone is looking to live longer, but almost no one wish to do anything about it. He was supported by Allen, who already observed the public ignorance in regards with LLSC Internet site. People are not interested in the theory of immortality, but maybe someone would be interested in practice of immortal life.

After several months we received first contact over the network, that confirmed one person starts the eternal life and could communicate with us. We were happy to know it. Some other people also contacted us, and it concluded the success of our publication.

The idea about immortality worked, and we can continue publishing our results.

Immortality and Eternity

Immortality relates to eternity but doesn't conclude it. Immortal life means living forever without dying, and eternity means elevating your spirit to the highest level the possible.

You can't live immortal life without constant perfection of your body and spirit, but you could elevate your spirit being mortal person. The history knows highly spiritual people who lived mortal life and don't intend to live forever. Moreover, some spiritual leaders reject the idea about immortality, and teach how to die consciously to get better afterlife.

We will not draw the conclusions about which way of life is better for people and let them decide. Our view on humans' destiny in Universe is based on accepting immortality as the most valuable form of humans' existence.

Immortality means living in heaven on Earth, but not in afterlife. Heaven on Earth is our vision of life, and not the geographical place on Earth with good climate.

Immortals accepting regular life as a special gift of god, and enjoy it as being in heaven. Life behind curtains, artificial walls and images, can be boring, senseless, and dull for mortal people. Eternity opens the way to immortality, and life becomes changed for better.

Each mortal person, who makes first step on the way to eternity, who decide to become immortal, already is immortal.

Aging and Dying Immortals

We were shocked by knowing that some immortals become sick, aged and, finally died. Does it crush our theory about immortal living? What was wrong?

Allen call me with this news and we came with Anthony and Allen together, to discuss this unfortunate discover.

Anthony smiled as usually, Allen was switched off, meditating on the reason of failed immortality, and I was tossing the news in my mind.

Did they fail the immortal life? If yes, then what part of it?

Three people was reported sick, one was dead and two other experienced significant loss of the personal energy.

Anthony first broke the silence and expressed his opinion on the news. He was sure that the theory is good, but some immortals didn't follow it as required and stay mortal at the certain time.

Allen turned his face to Anthony, but his eyes didn't see him.

"What you mean by this?" – He asked.

"Some rules where broken, and mortal people believed that they live immortal life, but it wasn't indeed" – was Anthony's answer.

I mentioned, that the theory of immortality does not include rules that regulate the mortal or immortal stage, it happens by itself when person is going from one stage to another.

Allen, finally, comes out of meditation and supports me by concluding that the theory is not guarantee the longevity, if person doesn't follow the body requests, then there is not changes from mortal to immortal person.

"People can honestly believe that they live the immortal life, but they are mortal instead" – concluded Allen – "intensions without actions does not conclude the result".

"Is anything that we can do with it?" – asked Anthony.

"Yes, we should be more precise by describing the stages of immortality" – was the Allen answer.

I was agreed with it, and we decided to work towards elaboration the details about stages in immortal life.

"What you suppose to write to the people?" – He asked, - "Something like, please be sure that you are immortal, otherwise you could age, suffer, and die, isn't it?"

We all laugh none regards to the serious situation. Really, how one can be sure that he is immortal by following the recommended procedures? We should give the explicit descriptions indicating that person is living immortal life, otherwise the entire teaching could mislead people, and cause unfortunate sequences that some already experienced.

What could be such regulations that can identify the fact that person is successfully changed life from mortal to immortal?

We talked to each other during about two hours without coming to the clear solution. There were several approaches to resolving the problem, including formal description of what changes in person could conclude the change from mortal life to immortal, practical examples of what happens in most immortal people by changing to eternal existence, and using internal vision for self-assessment.

All approaches require personal experience, good knowledge of theory, and extensive practice. How to assure anyone that his or her skills are enough to indicate the personal status of immortality?

Finally, we came to resolution, that mortal people are not able to indicate the stage of immortality. There is the circle of dependency where mortality can't be used to diagnose the immortality. System cannot evaluate itself without being elevated on a new level. Only immortal people can feel that mortality is gone.

We seated silently after coming to the point of conversation, when solution can't be found to be recommended to anyone.

Suddenly, Allen stood and said solemnly, that there is no contradiction with the theory of immortality, at all. The eternal life concludes the quality of human's life, but not the longevity. Immortal person is not dying because of style of life, and only the style of life must be accounted.

The meeting was ended with conclusion, that we are giving people the most luxurious life ever possible, that saves people life, but not concluded only eternal existence. People who safer with energy loss could not be considered as living immortal life, none regards to what they imagined about themselves.

Each of us decided to create the measurement scale that can be used for self-assessment the status of mortal person, who is changing to immortal being.

After several days we have met again to discuss the results and create the assessment requirements for the first stage in personal transition from mortal life to immortal.

The stage was named as "Departure", that means departing from mortal life to immortal. During this stage mortal person performs certain actions that must change the life. Allen's theory includes detail description of this stage, but we decided to add more descriptive indicators that can help people in self-assessment.

My Departure Stage

The goal of self-assessment is the measurement of how happy person is. Where are his feelings, believes, goals, emotions, and ideas on the way to joyful life?

The stage of mortal life, when the most negative symptoms are gone, could be concluded as change of immortal life. This system must assure the success in monitoring the life change, and segregate the real immortality from simply imagined longevity, when person honestly believe in living immortal life, but following mortal habits.

False immortality could produce temporary spikes in personal energy that can be wrongly assessed as signs of immortal life, but in longer range of time, the personal energy could go down and expose the signs of mortality.

Assuming all of this, the internal assessment must be permanent and practiced on all stages of eternal life.

"People must know the truth about themselves, otherwise tragic end will be achieved" – concluded Allen.

We shared our ideas with immortals over the network and found the absolute support from them.

On the first stage of immortal life all of us are still mortal and wish to change to immortal life. Strong desire starts the biological program hidden in our genes. It is a crucial, but not sufficient moment for change. Each of us must understand that successful change depends on our actions, and not based only on our "feeling good about immortality". Actions are required by our physical body and mind.

Changes happen in cells, tissues, blood, lymph, glands, bones, nerves, and everywhere. How to diagnose the success in changes?

Your overall feeling is better every day. Your movements, posture, walking style, balance, etc. becomes improved constantly.

Here is the part of the schema that Allen offered as the measurement scale for evaluation the signs of immortality, or the "level of immortality" in the mortal life.

The schema covers four main levels of human's life, including physical, emotional, intellectual, and social levels.

Physical level.

Body and mind are changing invisibly and constantly, that must be assessed each moment of your life to see the large picture of yourself and know where you are in your joyful immortal life.

Here is an example of what I assess and why.

1. My overall feeling can be assessed in form: "Am I happy? Do I feel the joyful bhoga (sweet feeling) flooding my cells? Are the dark and stressed cells, or group of cells, in my body? Is my entire body and cells bright?" I can conclude that my immortal life is not confirmed, if my positive feelings are not present, or negative feelings are identified. The correction of negative feelings is the next step in assessment. I am checking the meridians on the skin, and under the skin by watching it and changing dark colors to bright. This correction should change negative feelings in positive to affirm immortal life.
2. The second level of assessment includes evaluation the feelings in my head. "Do I feel any uncomfortable changes in my head?" I use the Energy Circle exercise to energies and restore blood flow in head, if I feel discomfort in it.
3. My neck will be the next level for evaluation. I perform energizing, or yoga, in case, if negative feelings or pain is in my neck, and newer leave it uncured.
4. The upper chest is the next in my assessment. I use my internal vision to examine cells in thyroid gland, and lungs.
5. The middle chest is the next in assessment. I am checking the heart, blood vessels, if any build ups are on the internal surfaces, and imperfections in valves. I use my energy to resolve any imperfection by concentrating the energy flow in the pace with damage. I also asses any muscles contractions are in veins and resolve it by warming up with my personal energy. I am checking the lungs in the middle part to remove any accumulations, or dark places. On this stage I also observe the color of my lungs to make it bright.
6. The lower part of the chest is the next part of self-assessment. I am checking the stomach, breathing membrane, lungs, liver, pancreas, lymph vessels, meridians, etc.

Dark, contracted, or painful zones need to be fixed by the concentration the personal energy on it.

7. The abdominal zone is the next in the self-assessment and includes evaluation of guts, gallbladder, kidneys, meridians, etc. The concentrated energy flow dissolves the dark clouds around some cells, if any.

8. Right hand and left hand are evaluated in the same way, and the difference is only in the meridians assessment. Different active zones on meridians are reacting differently on the energy flow. Sometimes I am using my palms to activate the energy flow where it is required.

9. Same procedure can be used for legs assessment. The special care should be given to feet, where the large number important energy flows are located.

10. Check the overall image of the personal energy. It should be evenly shaped in form of egg, or sphere. The outer age of personal energy should go out of your body boundaries, and not cross arms or legs.

11. Check the color of vital energy in shorter proximity to the body. The color must be evenly formed, white, with silver shine. This energy layer is going about ten or twenty inches out of your body.

12. Check the density of the personal energy. It must be like fur formed by tiny strings of energy joined together. This layer must be flexible, slightly resistant to pressure, and restores itself being stable in time. Make sure that your personal vital energy has no damaged form, density, or color. Sick people are surrounded by damaged energy with dark zones, not even form, and oily, liquid like, or "dusty" surface. Energy circle should be used to fix damages in vital energy before it will damage my body over the time.

13. Check my posture, movements, body position when seat and raise, check the voice strength and sound. My voice must be clear, sounds pleasant, and vibrating in resonance with my energy. I keep my body straight, move as fast as possible, but without rushing or impatience. I control my movements from the top point of my mind, and never let to be disoriented.

14. My fingers, palms, arms and legs performing well coordinated synchronous movements, being under control of Vipassana meditation.

15. All the above cannot be done by interruption my everyday living activity. All assessment is done in meditation that I am keeping in my mind and do it automatically.

16. The self-assessment becomes my habit that is same as breathing, or walking.

17. My constant control of the physical energy gives me joyful feeling of myself being logical and necessary part of the world. I feel that I am always in the best place and do my best in my life. I love the world and I am getting same feeling in return, being in harmony with the entire world. This feeling concludes the resonance with the Universal Energy.

18. I am checking my fast movements, that are not harmful to people, or objects, and not create discomfort to anything or anyone. I control, how I am holding glass of water, and bringing it as fast as possible in another room. The surface of water in the glass must be

flat, without spills or waves. I am keeping balance by riding in the municipal transport and loading weight only on feet, and not touching handles.

19. I am exposing myself to cold and hot weather without discomfort or pain. My personal energy works like a shield preventing me from the extreme environment. It gives me the luxury to be outside in any weather condition instead of hiding in shelters.
20. My food is always prepared in the way that I like, and it gives me the joy of nourishing myself. I observe the variety of available food by my internal vision and my body is shoving me what is my choice. I can cook special meal or buy it in the store, if I feel the necessity in it. Some of my food is in favor in my family, and I cook to the entire family.
21. My rule is that nothing can be on my plate that I can't eat separately such as spices, salt, sugar, vinegar, mustard, meat, etc. Apple cider mixed with water is an exception from it.

Emotional Level

Immortality is always associated with highly emotional acceptance of the world that is related to resonance that exists between us and the nature. Emotions are rich in variety, but flat in the volume. Beauty assumes the love and admiration of object of the interest. Love associates with emotions that sprinkles the hormones in the blood making our life joyful. Our brain can generate negative emotions when the personal energy is low and can't protect us from the changing world.

Negative emotions activate muscles activity and reduce the mental sharpness by preparing us to fight with imagined enemy. Bad, or negative, emotions are the symptom of insufficient energy. Emotional status can be assessed by us in the same way as we do it for physical body.

1. I am watching my emotions and classify it as good or bad. Good emotions mean love, passion, care, and bad emotions mean hate, anger and fear. When my emotional balance is changing, I try to understand and classify the reason of it. In the same time, I am checking the color of the emotional layer in my energy. This layer is the next after the vital energy and extends about twenty to forty inches out of body.
2. Pink color of energy means love to the sexual partner and constitute good energy. Same color, but with dark red flame means jealous, and bad energy. Dark red with black and gray flame means hate and anger that are signs of low energy.
3. The emotional layer is changing fast and protects the vital energy from disturbances. The early deficiency in personal energy can be diagnosed long before the vital energy becomes changed. It gives the immortal people the power of prediction any changes in the Universe.
4. Immortals are keeping slightly pink color with tint of yellow gold in emotional level. It looks like color of raised sun. I am checking this layer constantly to divert any disturbances from myself.
5. Life is variable and bad accidents happen everywhere. People grieving, being in emotional pain, suffer from loss, losing mind of irreversible events, and all of it substantially changing our emotional layer. Immortals suffer in the same way as all

mortals but recover much faster being cured by strong personal energy. Love to the entire world safes us from loss and suffer.

6. Vital energy is related to the emotional energy and they support each other being in harmony. People become sick being in emotional distress and become emotionally stressed being sick. Preventing bad emotions is important for prevention the person's vitality.

7. I am performing Vipassana and Energy Circle when my emotions are bad. The source of bad emotions can be easily found and resolved. I can't fix my bad emotions with insufficient personal energy. Mortal people simply don't pay attention to bad emotions, or even support it to demonstrate the "personal power" or looking for public understanding.

8. Negative emotions work like a bomb that destroys mortal body. Immortal people can't expect the longevity by experiencing negative emotions.

9. I need to understand the root of negative emotion and perform the meditation on it. Emotions with open roots becomes weak and are the subject for removal. I perform the combination of physical exercises, and Vipassana meditation on the bad emotions to eliminate it. The complete elimination can be achieved by repeated actions during the extensive time.

10. Elimination the bad emotions looks like removing weeds from the garden soil. It must be done periodically to let the good emotions to flourish.

11. My growing consciousness let me to understand the world with many relations in it. This knowledge helps me in deactivation wrong program in my mind and remove bad emotions from it.

12. Here is the practical example how my consciousness was used to diminish fear of people committed crime.

    We are surrounded by mortals that committed crime every day, and every minute, that based on dishonesty, cheating, stilling, abusing, forcing, killing, torching, seducing, tempting, refusing, denying, having affair, etc. These crimes may touch you directly or indirectly, but, no matter how you become aware about crime, it is against your vision of normal people behavior and could trigger repulsing feeling and negative emotion. How to convert this negative emotion in good feeling of love? Can we possible love something that is sharply against our vision of goodness in this world?

    The answer is "yes" for immortal people who can see the crime as the normal behavior of people with damaged personal energy.

    Are you angry of person who cannot run fast? Are you fear of people who is looking very old and ugly? Are you jealous of people who can swim faster than you?

    Probably, not, since you understand your position in this world, and the reason why the people are not the same as you are.

    Same thing is for the other people who demonstrate the ability to survive without producing socially requested values but grabbing this values from other people who work hardly to create it. We afraid and disgust of poisoned snakes, when we see it in the grass before us, but admire its beauty in the zoo, when they are in glass box. Our emotions protect us from the danger.

Immortals do not value the subjects of crime, and, consequently, do not feel bad emotions in regards with people who committed crime.

Immortals understand the wrong doing of mortals grabbing things from other mortals, and not support them in it, but don't feel bad about the crime, being outside of the crime zone.

Practice the Energy Circle exercise to eliminate bad feeling about anything in this world. Bad emotions constitute your detachment from the Universal energy that causes your aging.

Immortals should be careful with bad emotions and constantly assess the personal energy to eliminate it.

Intellectual Level

The third level in your personal energy relates to your intellectual activity, and involves the entire body in intellectual work, and not only your brain.

What is the work of brain? All what we do, is the result of brain activity implemented in the entire body actions. Intellectual work is related to emotions and vital activity.

Third level is extended from human's body further after the emotional level on about forty to sixty inches. The color of this level is unstable and reflects the brain and body activity being slightly blue, green, or yellow. Blue color reflects the logical activity in resolving some situations and making decision. Yellow color means actions with care about anyone or anything. The green color relates to the combination of both activities. Each color is good, if it is even, and bright. Uneven color, or dark color means hesitation in making decision, and mental deficiency.

Mental sharpness mixed with good intensions gives bright greenish color with blue hue.

I am assessing my intellectual level on the base of following symptoms.

1. I can perform math calculations in my mind. I try to not use calculators, or computers to perform simple calculations. My brain likes exercises and requesting me to perform some quizzes, tests, resolving problems, prove math equations, meditate on some math tasks, etc.
2. Good way in training memory is memorizing people's faces and names, and later restore names from my memory. I try to memorize the text that I read and repeat it. I try to restore in my memory the parking place where I placed the car, and how other cars were parked around my car.
3. The internal vision can be used to observe the places where I was and find something that I lost.
4. I use my memory not in a way as computer uses its memory, but as the media, that connects me to the Universe, where all information is located. It gives me the power to

see and know things that are far away from me in space and time. Some immortals reported that they use memory that gets an information from the "air".

5. Memory reverse view - is one of the best way to elevate my personal energy. I restore events in backward to see what happens with me in the past.
6. Activating brain during the sleeping time is also good exercise that gives the power to control uncontrolled intellectual activity. Simply, meditate on the waking up in your sleep, and once you will be able to do it.
7. I am planning more exercises that can improve my vision of the personal energy, including fast reading, parallel data processing, and learning new languages.

Social Level

This is the most outer level in the personal energy, and it extends farther over the sixty inches out of body. This energy supports your external activity, including communication with people, animals, plants, minerals, and other cosmic objects.

The social level is the most unstable level in my personal energy and it is related to intellectual, emotional, and vital levels. This level represents me to the entire world, and the world accepts me in regards with this level.

Immortal people should tune all internal levels to maintain good external level.

From the other hand, the social level can destroy lower levels, if misused. All four levels in human's personal energy are the fortress for protection the core of human being.

The structure of human's personal energy is one of the most complex in Universe, but it is almost the toy being compared with the structure of the Universal Energy, that is billions of times more advance than our energy. We call it "god".

The power of Universal energy is in its ability to generate more complex energies than it is now. This energy is growing in time and in space challenging us by its beauty and infinity. We try to resonate with the Universal Energy, but it is the same that run after the airplane.

We will never reach the complexity of the Universal energy, but we can constantly improve our personal energy to be in resonance with Universe as much as we can.

The complexity of personal energy is growing in geometrical proportion: each new level creates many new levels, and it expands like a blast. The growing personal energy doesn't only mean the increasing volume, but it means also the higher density and brighter color.

Personal energy is multileveled hierarchically built structure of energy pipes vibrating in resonance with each other and Energy of the Universe. Personal energy is also the shield protecting us from destruction. The probability of human's existence is higher than 75% and can go close to 100% when we are in the complete resonance with other energies. This movement is highly prized by our brain that discharges chemicals in our blood giving us the feeling of extreme joy and love.

In the moments, when the resonance is none perfect, the probability of our existence becomes lower than 100% and we feel it as exhaustion, weakness, or sickness. Lower probability means worse feeling and could cause illnesses by dropping around 80%-75%.

People, with significant destruction of the personal energy with probability around 75%, could attempt suicide having feelings that life has no meaning, and they can't keep the personal integrity, falling apart on simple components.

The resonance with the Universal Energy is not going automatically and requires control that my brain takes over the time of constant practice.

I can lose control over the personal energy, being in deep meditation, but always keep kind of side control on it, in case if personal energy drops. The stage of the energy control from the top of your attention named "Turiya".

Each new enhancement of my personal energy gives me a joyful feeling of "eureka". At the same time stage of Turiya becomes higher and can observe more structures in my energy. It means that I can better control my body and mind.

The moment of eureka is difficult to reach by simply planning it. It happens often occasionally, and I feel like my mind is ready for something, that I need to give the freedom to my mind to follow his actions. Suddenly, several meanings are joined together producing the new meaning that was previously never existed in my mind. My immediate eureka joy is converted in "...how could I never think about it?" feeling.

New idea could create a chain of related ideas going in the space of the brain that needs more energy to be penetrated. My next attempt is to resume the meditation on these ideas again, but it not always possible since my energy may be not enough to keep my resonance on it.

The watch point Turiya remembers the entrance to the secret zone and will guide me in the next time. The very short moment between feeling of approaching eureka and enlightening with new idea is measured by several seconds, or even shorter than second. We call this moment "Prajna", or the moment before knowing something. Prajna takes a lot of energy to display image on our senses to be understood.

Body Calls

The immortal body's wish is named as "body calls". We must respect our body calls and satisfy it.

In the beginning of immortal life, I received two types of body calls, related to my mortal and immortal life. Each type of body calls could require different actions, and I try to segregate one type from another.

My regular mortal desire was related to continuation the mortal life in form of rejecting extra activity, exercises, and meditation. Mortal life is, usually, associated with low energy and rejects action associated with high energy.

Mortal body calls can request me to act against my wellbeing by suggesting skipping the exercises due to the lack of the time, go later to bed due to the interesting TV show, or news, eat food overloaded by calories to feel "full stomach", demonstrate my negative emotions to "protect myself", suppress the rights of the other people on the behalf of my own rights, punish someone, because I was insulted by someone, etc.

Immortal body calls are different, and let you feel uncomfortable to ignore it. The immortal internal "voice" is quiet and gentle, but very persistent and exists until satisfied. The example of immortal call can be: perform certain exercises, yoga poses, food, air, water, get sunlight, be in seawater, perform breath exercises, do meditation, read certain books or articles, sing certain songs or sounds, etc.

The immortal body calls can overflow your ability to perform all of it in the beginning of your immortal life. It happened with me, when immortal life unfolds in form of powerful energy flow during the week after starting the immortal program.

I was ready for immortal living due to my developed personal energy, and my mind accepted the idea of eternal living without any hesitations. I know that Allen started his immortal living much earlier than the rest of us, and he shared his experience with us, expecting our critical feedback.

We accepted his story without any skepticism, because we were ready for it. Each of us worked with human's longevity and was familiar with methods and technics. Immortality is the process of continuous longevity, and nothing else, except the fact that longevity is not starting the immortal program in us but prepares us to it.

The start point of immortal life is important, as the key for changes. The moment, when I consciously decided that I am immortal, and watched myself in the following minutes, hours and days, was very important to me. It was my secret that I kept several months, before to reveal it to my family.

What I was waited for? I wish to enjoy the secrecy of my changes, to play with my ego and boost my expectations. It is, probably the secret that anyone enjoy by getting something extraordinary in they life.

Members of my family react differently on my immortality. My wife becomes a bit scared and angry on me. My kids were prepared for my extraordinary habits and react moderately.

The relation between us gradually become the same as it was before, but my immortality was cited mostly for fun, until I become changed in better way. My changes shift the family mood to the side of acceptance, as it is now. No one followed the immortal life habits, but some healthy rules were accustomed and practiced.

I remember my first immortal calls that sounds periodically in me. It was call to jog in the park that is close to my house. The call was so much strong, that I surrender to it, and run as fast as I can, having heart bit, and tiredness almost diseased me in first several minutes. The immortal call was happy and suggested me to reduce the pace and run as I feel joyful. It resolved the problem, and I was the happiest person in the world. The immortal call says: "You are very good".

The next body call was about weight lifting and pooling body up. I am not an athlete, and never performed such things before. In the books I found what needs to be assembled to satisfy my immortal body call. Over the time I built the pool-up construction on my backyard and attached the weights to it.

The reaction on my attempts to pool-up myself, and lift the weights was very positive, but my skills in it was very poor, until I repeat exercises during several months.

Internal calls were never stop and requested me to wear only shorts to perform exercises on my backyard, no matter what is the weather. I accepted these calls, and the next immortal voice requested me to stop eating meat to protect myself from getting cold being outside.

I wasn't heavy meat eater, but this strict request surprised me, and a bit disappointed, since I surely need proteins to build muscles.

I know that I must follow immortal calls, and I cut the meat consumption. The miracle happens soon after when the cold winter with temperature falling lower twenty degrees Celsius, and I was exercising on my backyard.

My feet become frozen badly, and I didn't feel it about fifteen minutes after coming back in the room. The skin on feet was peeled off soon, and I decided to wear sandals if the temperature is lower than ten degrees Celsius.

I didn't contract any cold and feel fresh and happy being outside in deep frost with strong wind.

The next call requested me to reduce the water temperature in shower after I finished washing my body. It was harder to perform than to exercise on the frost. Cold water makes me change my energy, muscles tension, and deep breathing.

Body calls teach me to visualize my internal body cells when I am experiencing some changes in body. Once in a morning, I feel heaviness in the right side of my abdominal and think of what it could be. The immortal voice immediately gives me advice to "watch" inside of the feelings. I did what was recommended and found an image of the contracted pipe that has some dark content in it. Voice recommended to send the hot white energy in the dark place to relax the zone and restore the guts movement. I concentrate my attention on what was suggested, and visualize the dark zone becomes lighter with unpleasant feelings ended at the same time.

Body calls can be compared with the "Angels Voice" described in ancient books, and in the Bible. I think, that it is the same, but I don't believe in angels, and believe in my own consciousness that guides my being immortal. The immortal calls are the way, how immortal program unfolds in my body.

Eternal body calls are even more interesting in the resolving my emotions that are more difficult to manage. "Be careful with your anger, you are shifting to mortal being now" – is the internal message, that I cannot ignore, and my anger disappears immediately.

"I have to be more attentive to the mortal people to help them." – was call in my mind. It was the mortal body call that assumes my superiority and it was the sign of my energy decline. The energy circle exercise was required to fix it.

Any ideas about myself being special, or miserable, was rejected by my immortal body calls. My importance means nothing in this world, only the personal energy is valued.

On the stage of Departure, I often compare myself with other people acknowledging the difference. Each time, when I do it, I was penalized by my immortal energy. The immortal calls stated: "I am losing my attention, destroying my resonance, spreading my energy in unnecessary actions. People are perfect as they are, don't fool yourself by thinking about your superiority, you are on the wrong way. You could compare yourself with the other people, if you become mortal again".

In the beginning of my immortal life, I got different body calls, related to my brain activity. One of such call was the request for balance of multiple processes acquiring simultaneously. Juggling with stakes and balls were only one side of the immortal calls. I was required to perform several independent actions in the same time that pushed my brain in extreme state.

Immortal calls often challenged me to go out of boundaries of mortal life by performing actions, feeling, and thinking differently. Immortal program in my body crushed my mortal comfort by imposing strange and unreasonable requirements on me, such as exposing to cold weather, fasting, performing strange physical exercises, that look like yoga, but not the same as am doing every day.

Sometimes, I blindly follow the body calls without delay, but in some cases, it takes time to satisfy the body calls. I guess, that I couldn't satisfy it all. My effort in body calls satisfaction ends up with more waves of calls, and it never stops.

The complexity of immortal calls is also rising. The resonance with Universal energy requests me to be ready for larger extend.

Once, being in a car and listen to classic music, I realized, that choral songs sound like the Universal sound, that I couldn't reproduce by combining the sounds of different musical instruments, or electronic vibrations. Choral singing in churches activates the vibrations in personal energy and helps in establishing the resonance with the Universe. Singing and listening is important for us, and often requested by immortal program.

Immortal calls requesting me to learn how to play the musical instruments, singing, creating the music, looking on synchronicity in different musical fragments, manipulating with my voice, and making it sound exactly as musical notes. Resonance in music, emotions, voice, and meanings, was one of my priority in satisfaction immortal calls with physical activity together.

I was shay to sing on public, and made my voice exercises on my kitchen, or car, instead. The immortal voice suggests, that sound of my voice should go inside of me, but not outside. It was difficult to understand the inversion of my voice inside myself, but, over the time, I was learned it, and now I can sing at any place without the problem.

In singing, the vibration of singer's body, is more important, than the song produced for other listeners. I can't keep my voice complete silent for the people and sing when the air is saturated with other sounds to keep my vibrations hidden.

One of the interesting body call was the attention to the skin. I have never pay attention to my skin and was a bit surprise why such immortal call was issued to me.

The skin is part of us that is visible for our eyes, and tangible by our fingers. It is very much accessible organ that can be evaluated and changed.

I found that my skin has a lot of imperfections, including pigmented spots, wrinkles, scars, tiny buildups, etc. The immortal calls suggested to use the meditation to improve the skin condition.

The surface of skin is significant, and I didn't know how I can use meditation to deal with my skin.

My skin has billions of thin canals, connected to the layers assembled in the skin. My skin appears the complex structure, that can't be considered as "leaser cover".

Immortal calls suggested to start from the inner layers of the skin, connected by energy pipes with the energy centers, and vital organs in my body.

Here I found uneven energy distribution in the lower skin layers and try to energies the dark and cold spots.

After several months of such meditation, my skin becomes smoother, and shinier.

Gradually I lifted the point of meditation on the upper level of my skin and found that wrinkles become less visible.

In the same time, I got some immortal calls, related to my diet and physical exercises. I didn't receive these calls before I start my mediation on the skin.

Skin displays our personal energy to us. Smooth, elastic, and shiny skin displays good personal energy, and grayish, uneven, and wet skin means the energy deficiency.

Skin is one of the most important organ in our body, that connects us with the outer world by breathing, perspiration, temperature regulation, protection from bacteria, absorbing water and minerals, activation the energy centers, mechanical protection, curing almost all diseases, etc.

Historically, all organs in our body comes from the skin, and tightly connected with it. Healthy skin means healthy body, and vice versa. Immortals are very concerned about the skin that extends our brain, making it connected to the Energy of the Universe.

The structure of the skin is much more complex, than we think, including special zones, where energy connects to the Universal energy pipes. We call it "meridians", that are ancient regulatory channels in human's body. Meditation on the energy in meridians makes our skin and body immortal.

You never know, what your immortal program will request from you to move your life on the next stage of immortality.

Immortal program that unfolds in our body breaks our mortal superstitions in the same way, as a bright sun and warm weather breaks the ice on the river, starting from several locations, and then breaks the ice everywhere.

Feeling of the Resonance

The resonance with Universal energy produces pleasant feeling in the entire body and is the source of immortal joyful life.

Feeling of dissonance is also very much noticeable, when your personal vibrations are not in resonance with the other vibrations. Dissonance creates unpleasant feeling of danger, unbearable discomfort of destruction of the personal energy, and losing the resonance with the Universe. Feeling of dissonance requires immediate escape from the "wrong" vibrations, or conversion it in "good" vibrations.

The "good" and "bad" vibrations can be produced by different people, news, music, art, meal, meanings, etc. Immortal calls requested me to learn how to convert "bad" vibrations in "good" one.

The conversion "bad" to "good" was so much difficult, as, for example, eating poisoned meal as the good one. The eternal voice was requesting me to accept what is bad as good. The goal of that call was not classifying world on bad and good but accept it as it is. Nothing is good or bad, but only vibrating Universe. The quality of vibration relates to the vibrating structure. Only my personal expectations could make me lover or hater. My personal schema of the world damages my vibrations and makes me being dependent on my own mistakes.

Immortal calls were very persuasive in clearing my acceptance of "bad" vibrations. Sometimes I feel free from "bad" vibrations, and experienced the complete freedom from it, being in perfect resonance with the Universe, but, sometimes, I fail it badly, and feel my strong dependency on it.

Surprisingly, my eternal voice didn't require my complete obedience to this request, and softly pushes me in right direction. It was one of the most difficult part of my departure period.

I try to involve my logic to find anything good in "bad", but it doesn't work. Then I try to "excuse" what is "bad" to accept it as "good", and it doesn't work either. Any attempts in reaching consent with "bad" vibrations were miserable failed until immortal voice suggests seeing "bad" as the component of "good". It takes a time, before I grasped the meaning of it. The "bad" was gone immediately at the time when my mind jumps on the next level of understanding, that we call "eureka".

The space without "good" and "bad" vibrations is a paradise. The heaviness of the world is gone, all dark places becomes lightened, and resonance with Universe feels like never stops.

How come, that I lived so many years being mortal? What stopped me from this joy in the past? I wish to take hands of mortal people and bring them here, to show, what could be the life in the haven. How to get hands of people, if they are so far from me, living behind the walls of the illusions and false images?

I always wish to share my happiness with others, if I can. It is, probably, normal intension of any person, none regards with mortal status. I wish to show this luxurious life to others, but how to transfer feelings, if you are alone staying in the haven before the eternal Universe, and only single sparks of other souls are visible around, and silence of singularity is pressing on me slightly? The immortal voice is calling me to go far further from the feeling of joy, and get more excited any time, when new step is successfully accomplished.

Immortal joy newer stops but requires me to step up on the next level, where the previous level looks like nothing special. The joy of accomplishing the new level exceeds the joy of being on the same level, and it pools you to go up in your life. The resonance with the Universe is infinite, and newer be finalized, since the Universe is incomparably more complex than we are, and complexity of the Universe is growing in each moment in geometrical progression.

Constant progress in my personal energy gives me the feeling of eternal joy, that can be compared with mortal temporary feelings created by intaking the hallucinogens drugs.

Drugs destroy the personal energy by overproducing the neuro-mediators that makes people addictive to it. Immortal resonance makes my personal energy stronger without drugs or addiction.

On the late stage of the departure period, I was free from constant evaluation of my immortal life and compare myself with mortal people. Immortal life cannot be compared with mortal in any aspects, and immortals don't enjoy by feeling the superiority. It is no "superiority" at all, because, nothing can be compared, except the feeling of high joy. There are two incomparable styles of human's life, where people can't understand each other, in terms of the quality of life, but can live with peace and love to each other. Immortals love mortals and vice versa.

Mortals think about immortals as people, who live in fantasy and delusion being happy of themselves, and not creating problems for mortals. Mortals believe that immortals will die anyway.

Immortals feel strong desire to bring mortals to immortal world, and make them happy, young, and healthy. Immortals newer think about ever existence but would like to enjoy life forever.

Mortals newer think about immortal life as the most luxurious form of human's life, but always associate it with the living without death. It is understandable, since mortals have never experienced the immortal joy, and can't even approximately imagine this feeling. All what mortals can expect from immortal life is the longevity.

Immortals, on the other hand, rarely think about longevity, and mostly concentrate on the joyful life. Longevity comes by itself due to rejuvenated immortal body.

Feeling of the resonance with the Universe is associated with meditation that is normal stage of immortal life. The meditation here I associate with Turiya state of mind, or constant life supervision from the upper point of mental observation.

Immortal Meditation.

Meditation means the mental control and observation of main stages of my body-mind activity. Without such control, my life becomes spontaneous and uncontrollable like jumping molecules in an air. Outside of meditation, I can spend hours in rotating some ideas in my mind and break the resonance with the Universe.

Meditation is mandatory, and body calls will promote it in the first half of the departure period. Being in meditation, I am experiencing joyful feeling of mindfulness, and wholeness. It brings parts of me together and helps me in getting my entire body-mind in one place, in form of strong cosmic object that can vibrate in resonance with other objects.

I feel myself, as disassembled in parts, when I am losing my meditation, and I need a minute to come back to it. Meditation cleans mind and body, makes us younger and stronger.

In the beginning, I meditate by resolving my body calls, and started from the simple Vipassana.

This type of meditation is well known and affordable by anyone. Vipassana endorsed my consciousness to the Prajna, and I was mediating on it quite a long time, that is about two years. In the same time, I meditated before sleep to keep track of my night sleeping with dreams and without dreams. The success wasn't persisted even after several years of exercises, but substantially improved my ability to keep Turiya state, and accomplish some stages in Pratyahara.

Spontaneously, I am sliding in Dharana and Dhyana meditation, but wouldn't consider myself as experienced practitioner.

The highest form of resonance can be reached by being in high stage of Dhyana, and in Samadhi. The ecstatic feeling in Samadhi is the cosmic love to the Universe.

In the last stage of immortal life, that we call "joy", people are living in persistent Samadhi that concludes the name of this stage.

The Energy Circle exercise is based on Vipassana meditation, and includes Tratak, Pratyahara, Dharana, and Dhyana. All these mental practices, joined together, are the path to Samadhi.

I am not going to describe my effort in gaining the progress in the Energy Circle, each of us should go by our own way, but all these ways are coming together in one point, that is the resonance with Universal energy, or Samadhi.

It is always difficult to accomplish in the beginning of immortal life, but later, it becomes a regular habit, when resonance becomes unnoticeable and acquires by itself.

It is the same, as we see the sunlight, when we are going out of darkness, but later we don't pay attention to the bright sun.

I was newer in the perfect resonance with the Universe, since it always changes, and I try to adjust my vibrations to it. I am happy in the moments when I do my best, and my happiness changes in achieving feeling when my resonance becomes a bit dissipated. It looks like you drive on the street, and adjust your direction, to be in the middle between two lines. Most of time you do it successfully, but, in some cases, your position can be not so perfect, and you need to turn the steering wheel. You do it subconsciously, but always with attention (Turiya) on the road.

I started my Vipassana by sitting on the floor in my room with legs crossed, and arms rested on my knees. My first exercise was in watching my breath. I still performing this meditation in any situation, when I have difficulty to keep Samadhi.

My brain is not well trained yet, and sometimes it is going out of my supervision, and jumps up and down, as the young horse escaped to freedom.

I always laugh by watching it and let it to become tired before to impose Vipassana. My immortal calls didn't allow me to be tough on my brain and ask me to be gentle with it. I was satisfied of my eternal life and not planned to change it any time later.

In the end of the "departure" period in immortal life, I become completely accommodated to constant meditation, and can't even imagine myself existing with the uncontrolled mind.

I remember, when I feel myself a bit disintegrated, upset and heavy, only one word "resonance" in my mind immediately brings me in one piece together, making me happy again.

It was a remarkable feeling of bright hot light vibrating in my forehead, throat, heart, stomach, and abdominal, that link all together in hot cloud of energy. In the cold climate, where I live, it immediately protects me from being frozen.

Resonance protects me from extreme heat, when I travel in desert of Egypt. I use the energy circle when I feel that my Samadhi is not perfect, and I am going out of the resonance with the world.

In the moment, when my meditation is not deep enough, I feel that something wrong happens, and immediately check the resonance by assessing the feelings in my energy centers. My internal vision displays the gray clouds or dark dots in energy centers that must be eliminated by the vibrations. I start the energy circle that fixes the resonance, and I am becoming happy again.

The scenario above is usual for immortals on the early stages of departure period, and later, you become rarely upset, being mostly a happy person.

The ability of being in meditative stage in the most of your time is concluding the beginning of the second stage in your immortal life, when you are changing and becoming immortal person.

Changes in me weren't irreversible and were depended on my ability to be in resonance with cosmic energy. Good resonance brings remarkable changes, and pure resonance didn't contribute to positive changes.

My personal energy is changing up and down depends on the multiple conditions, including biological rhythms, work load, weather, and resonance with other energies.

I am losing my resonance when my energy is dropping lower than usual level, and I activate the energy circle immediately, when it happens. Losing the resonance associates with the feeling of something bad is going to happen soon, or the feeling of cold pressure in energy centers. It feels like fear of life.

Sometimes I am losing so much energy, that I can't restore it during several minutes, or even hours. In this case, I try to visualize the source of my energy loss, but it is rarely possible, since I am usually not being in resonance with objects consuming my energy. It could be someone, that I know, or someone, connected to me over the network. Such form of the energy share is not imposed on me intentionally by energy "vampires", but, possibly, is created spontaneously by people who is in trouble and need help. It could be one person with ability to communicate over the network, or the number of people who suffer by energy loss.

Occasional energy losses have been reported by many immortals, and we investigate this phenomena in our group. We found, that such energy loss happens due to the combination of several conditions, including instability of the personal energy and urgent request for energy sent over the network.

Normal, not violent, energy share is the process of establishing resonance with people who is requesting it. This resonance improves the personal energy of other people and positively contributes to the immortal energy.

In case, when the personal energy is unstable due to the natural causes, it could be spontaneously involved in resonance with unknown object, that creates problems to immortal being, that ends up with frustration, and sadness.

These unfortunate events happen with novices in the beginning of immortal life, and rarely possible later, when personal energy is strong enough to compensate external vibrations created by unknown sources.

Most of the time my resonance is good, and joyful sweet feeling is flooding my body. I am checking my resonance that is like the pilot checking the altitude in aircraft's cockpit.

All, what I described above, relates to the meditation in my awaking consciousness that contributes about seventy percent in my energy balance.

In the same time, the meditation in my sleep time is also important, and does the work, that is impossible to expect from meditation in awaking stage.

We sleep to restore our energy. The meditation during this time is important to make the restoration manageable and effective.

I ignored the last form of meditation, decided, that I should sleep and have a good rest, instead of stressing myself with meditation. It was a mistake, since meditation is form of release from stress, rather than impose it.

My first experience with night meditation connects with the practice of Yoga Nidra that prepares my mind to be in deep sleep with active Turiya. Yoga Nidra not assumes my sleeping stage, and, even, prohibits it, but, in my case, I use it to relax my mind to be able to enter it.

Later, after extended practice, I could recall the external sounds, and my physical movements during the sleep. I also was able consciously enter my night dreams and perform volunteer actions in it. My interesting observation was, that dreams become much more bright, colorful, and easily memorable, after I entered it. In my night dreams I could fly, move objects by the power of my will, go through the objects, see and talk to other people, etc.

Why it happens in the dreams? It is, probably, the reminder, that immortals can do it in awaking stage of the consciousness. My immortal friends told me, that it is possible, and I believe them.

The meditation at the sleep time is a bit different than meditation in the awaking mode. Part of our brain is newer sleep all the time, but accurately manages the body restoration process.

I feel that my skin becomes colder at evening time, and my energy is collapsing in the center of my body, causing drowsiness, losing attention to outside world, and fatigue. Right before to surrender to the sleep, I perform three deep breathes, and mentally write my wish in the center of my forehead about keeping my meditation during the entire time of sleep. Basically, I am asking my brain to extend Turiya to the night sleep.

It could happen that you will be able to manage your feelings in your sleep from the first attempt. I was not such a lucky person, and try many times, before to succeed.

My mortal friends can't understand, how I can be in meditation all the time, even when I sleep. They convince me, that meditation should consume all my mind, my attention, and nothing could be left for my everyday activity.

It partially correct, and, in the beginning, my mind was completely consumed by meditation. I was not able to do anything or think about anything when I meditate. Later I found myself meditating when I am walking, driving a car, waiting in line, talking and listening, eating, etc.

My meditation was like a cloud in my mind that condensed and moved back to the side clearing my consciousness for sharp vision and fast reaction.

Meditation cleans my mind in the same way as the aerosol spray cleans air by removing small particles from it. I would consider, that my meditation removes small circling ideas from my mind and gives me the time for better concentration on one or two of it.

The mind of immortals can process several tasks simultaneously. Some immortals can perform parallel actions that mortals found difficult or barely possible to do. Parallel reading, speaking, writing by both hands, memorizing visual and logical information, etc.

My immortal body calls request me to exercise the simultaneous actions, math calculations being processed in mind with no records, and memory training.

These calls are very much persistent, as calls for physical exercises.

How our immortal mind knows, what we need to do to be immortal? This information is written in codes of the internal program that runs my immortal mind. I have never think about many of the exercises that body-mind calls have requested me to perform.

It is fun to satisfy immortal calls, and it gives the result, that improves my life. My memory becomes sharp, and I can recall such details, that I would never consider is possible for me. My reaction becomes fast, and I can move much faster, simple for fun and pleasure. Performing several tasks in parallel is also kind of pleasure, and time saving habit.

My meditation is also changing over time. In the beginning I was seating in classic yoga pose, and perform Vipassana, now my meditation comes to the point when I can concentrate my attention on my energy moving around my body cells, and in other objects. In meditation I can mentally talk to other objects having contact with, practically, anything in the world.

I feel the same as other objects feel, and it makes me closer to these objects. Mortal society traditionally divides world on two sides, where one side is living entities, and the other side is none living objects. Mortals see living objects, as something, that can feel, react on the world, replicate each other, and support the integrity. Immortals see the "none living objects" as the same that "living" objects. All objects are the part of one living Universe and can't be divided in any way.

My mortal friends ask me to compare the stone with the bird, where stone is "dead", and bird is "alive". I asked them to describe the difference in these two objects, and, as a result, no difference has been found, since both are moving, replicating, growing, consuming, changing in time, etc. The entire world has been created by the same scheme, as the vibrating energy pipes, bended in nodes. Any attempts in dividing this world on groups, will not succeed.

I found for myself, that removing classifications from objects is the same as removing curtains from the windows. It opens the sun of knowledge come in the dark room of superstitions.

My meditation is changing from the partial analysis of objects to the integration objects in the entire Universe. Each my small step gives the feeling of "eureka", and the world becomes wider and brighter. It can be compared with hiking, when new steps extend the horizon.

In the beginning of immortal life, my mind requested the meditation, as the result of body-mind calls, and later, the meditation by itself requested my mind to resolve the immortal calls. Meditation became the form of my mind's vision of the world.

Without meditation, I can't see the integrity of the world, but only it parts in the mist of uncertainty. One image is mixing with other, and, it becomes closed by my mental phantasy, that creates the illusory environment where ordinary people are living mortal life.

Having the experience with advance meditation, I perform simple Vipassana five minutes exercise in each morning, to keep my skills sharp, as requested my body calls.

The time disappears, when I perform Vipassana, and I become fresh and active during the entire day.

I would say, that meditation is the number one immortal exercise for me. It accompanies all other my exercises, making it pleasurable.

Mortals are not accepting immortal world, since it doesn't exist for them. They simply denying it and don's bother to accommodate to it. The different story is with immortal people who are living in immortal world and communicate with its mortal illusion created by mortals.

I remember emotional days when I started my immortal life and elevated my personal energy a little. I was so much happy, that can't resist to share this tremendous news with others. I was alone with my happiness, as a stranger in the forest. I feel my isolation until the time when the network becomes accessible, and I can share my feelings with other immortals.

I can meet my friends at work, but they feel differently, or the same, being immortal by themselves. We share the same ideas, being isolated in our small immortal group. Allen and Anthony were first who contacted the network, and I was the last in our group.

Every day I try hardly to become connected, but it was out of my effort, and I surrendered to the nature of myself, and decided to be with myself ignoring my failure.

The contact with the network comes by itself, as it was described by Allen and Anthony, without any attempts from my side. I simply become connected and see other immortals as clearly as they see me.

Long time ago I was living my mortal life, like being in the theatre of illusions, believes, artificial rules, none existed danger, and precautions. I can't believe, that all this unreal world, can be created by the natural humans' evolution. How come, that my mind knows different world, that simply exists in the parallel immortal space on the same location as the mortal world? Am I a prisoner of my own fantasy, or I can feel something that mortals can't feel?

The network helped me in getting answers on my questions, and I understand, that I my world is not the fantasy, but the normal reality, that looks like fantasy being compared with mortals' vision.

The simplicity of immortal world surprised me more, than the complexity of mortal world. I told many times to myself, that I could be wrong in getting all surrounded world as the part of myself, instead of hanging curtains and names on objects to divide it from each other. My scientific consciousness was against the artificial classification and segregation the objects on parts, it didn't work for me, I stopped to understand the reality. I see data, collected in tables, curves, and diagrams, conclusions, and opinions, different meanings of the same, that has only one meaning. We debated, discussed, created schemas and plans of simple things that do not require it due to the simplicity of its origin and its existence. Basically, we mentally circle in our own illusions to create more illusions and be proud of its complexity. World is simple and immortal. Mortality begins from the attempts to describe the world by using illusions, or, my lovely word: "hypotheses". The idea of hypothesis is, to create mortal stamp on the objects that artificially removes it from the connection with other objects to investigate as separate entity. This is the root of mortality.

Nothing can be separated, named, imprisoned in research boundaries, and subjected to opinion in immortal world. All is one, and one is all in the real immortal world.

As an example, I cannot effectively manage the energy in my heart without tuning energy in my liver, kidneys, abdominal zone, and many other centers inside and outside my body. We are not living in isolated world, all is united, pulsing and communicating.

If I am in a good mood, then it means, that all my cells, and people around me are in good connection. The illness means the energy destruction in the entire body and around the ill person. If some surgeon cuts off "bad" cells from human's body to cure the illness, then it violates the idea of immortal life, and the integrity of the human's body, that will cause the illness to come back again. Sick person must change they life to cure the disease.

Mortal medical doctors will give you procedures or medications, instead of providing the adequate energy treatment. Behind the curtains of illusion and fantasy, the ill person will safer of illness, until self-recover, or die.

The integrity of the nature is the subject of biocenosis, and ecology. The illusion of independency vanishes, as soon as you become immortal person, and able to see the world without curtains.

I was on the stage of curiosity in relations between mortal and immortal world, when my personal energy becomes a bit elevated. It was a normal feeling of the superiority, when energy is not weak, but is not strong enough to give a clear vision of things.

Mortal people like to be outside of the large towns to touch and admire of the nature. It is the instinctive attachment to the real immortal world that is not hidden behind the multiple curtains, schemas, and superstitions.

Connection with natural objects creates the resonance with these objects and improves the personal energy. Mortals become quickly tired, being in the contact and resonance with the nature, and follow the regular routine by switching the attention to the lovely curtains.

Sometimes, I asked myself, are these curtains also the part of the nature? Why mortals are attached to it so much, that wasted huge amount of time to observe it?

The nature has been created as the result of the evolution, and mortal curtains and screens also are created as the result of human's evolution. It means that nothing wrong is in mortal detachment from one world and attachment to the other world. Why artificial human's world would be "wrong" and immortal Universe would by "right" for us? All of us mortal, and immortal are created by the same Universe and are living as the one entity.

The question is: can one entity be partially mortal and partially immortal?

My logic suggests, that this is impossible. I hope, that you agree with me. We all are inherently immortal by the birth but become mortal due to the isolation from the main source of the energy, like the cells in immortal body, that are dying constantly supporting immortal life.

We are not grieving about dying cells in our body, but we are immortal, because of this. Cells are not able to resonate with the Universe during the entire life and fix imperfections in its body. Resources of the energy will be exhausted, if not restored. Only human's intelligence knows how to resonate with Universal energy, being immortal.

Can animals be immortal? We can positively answer this question, if some animals will elevate the personal energy to the level of acceptance the immortal life.

The resonance with cosmic energy can be the main instinct in some animals, who possess the immortality and enjoy the beautiful life. Did you see these animals? Some could live in the deepness of the ocean, or hide in the wilderness, but they are connected to the network, as none human creatures, and we can contact them, being immortal.

Allen and Anthony often told me about none human creatures, who possesses significant personal energy to become accessible in the network. I couldn't see them, but believe my friends, that it is possible.

Once in my meditation I got a call from such a creature, who, presumable, was a large animal in the ocean. This animal talked to me with the wisdom of guru. I was shocked, and can't believe, that it happens in real, and wasn't my fantasy. This humanistic animal was huge in size, and I feel and see what was around this animal. The most impressive was the feeling of joy produced by this immortal being.

I didn't feel my superiority by contacting with other none-human objects in the Universe. They are everywhere and become visible during my meditation. Can I see it in the best movie I have ever seen, or read about it in a book, or meet such unusual thing in my dreams?

The contact with immortal creatures is not only observing the other life and other worlds, but the coexistence in similar feelings of joy, that can't be the result of fantasy, or imagination, but are the real emotions of coexistence in one Universe. It feels like we all are singing the same song that newer ends.

My immortal feelings suggest me that this first contact with multiple forms of immortality, is the first step towards the entire proliferation in cosmic life. This life is so much attractive and promising, that I feel the goosebumps on my skin by contacting it.

I shared my excitement with Allen, and he congratulated me with my successful movement further in the world of eternity. My amusement was mixed with uncertainty in my understanding of coexistence the highly changing Universe with immortality. I asked Allen about it.

Allen laughs, as usually, making jokes of my question. He said, that rigid things become broken, and flexible things stay as it is. The immortality is possible due to the changes in us, and we will die otherwise. Our cells are dying, consumed by other cells, and replaced in the same way, as our energy is replaced by the new personal energy that is more advance.

Flexibility and changes in the Universe is the form of immortal life. The Universe by itself is immortal and propagates this low on all its parts. The parts of the universe can be mortal, as the components of immortal objects. The difference between immortal and mortal objects is in the level of "understanding" of cosmic low. This "understanding" comes from the personal energy created on the base of the initial personal energy inherited by the birth.

Allen was right, the personal energy is the level of "understanding" of what is mortal, and how it can be used to support the immortality.

I asked Allen about our future. Can we expect, that our parts will become such intelligent entities, that possess they own immortality?

Allen said, that it will be our future. The unity of us will not be in jeopardy, since immortal parts are united in immortal being due to tight communication between parts. Or internal organs are, in fact, immortal under the influence of the personal energy.

Your liver restores itself being the part of you, but it will die, being separated from you. You restore yourself, being the part of the immortal entity, that is Earth, and you will die being separated from it. The Earth is an immortal part of the Solar System, but it will die, being separated from it. The Solar System is the immortal part of our galaxy but will die being separated from it. The world is inherently immortal as the part of other immortal systems connected in the endless Universe.

The immortal parts can become mortal, when the personal energy is dissipated, and immortal integrity becomes no longer possible. It means the death of mortal parts and consuming it by other immortal objects with high personal energy.

Allen stated, that this process is consistent and concludes the life cycle in the Universe.

Why immortal objects can become mortal? What brings the personal energy to the lower stage?

Allen always emphasized, that the difference between mortal and immortal world is the illusion. It is not such curtain that can be hanged in between two objects and name it "mortal" and "immortal".

The mortality is the stage of any object and depends on it current personal energy, and the ability to resonate with the rest of the world. Mortal object can become immortal for a moment, and then come back to mortal stage again. The same can happens with immortal objects.

Immortal life is the way to support immortality, and it not guarantee the immortality by itself. Immortality is the opportunity, rather than the condition.

Immortal person has an ability to improve the personal energy but naming themselves as "immortal" doesn't guarantee the immortality as a fact.

I constantly experience my energy come up and down, being in resonance with other energies. How can I be sure that I am Immortal?

Allen was excited of my selfishness and shortage of vision. He was curious, why I need to be sure, that I am immortal? Why you, really, need to be the one?

I was shocked by his questions, having in mind that all our activity is dedicated to proving, that immortality is possible, and can be offered to other people.

He said, that my vision is wrong, as I would never be immortal at all.

Why you are living immortal life? – He asked me.

I love it, it is joyful, absolutely incredible, new, entertaining, attractive – was my answer.

Now, you speak as immortal being – He said.

Immortality is the optimum form of life, when all energy is condensed in body cells and managed to become better each single moment of our life. Therefore, you feel that your energy comes up and down, because you care about it, and because you are immortal being.

Immortality can be broken, if the personal energy is not strong enough to take care about itself. It means the end of the object's integrity.

It could happen with people, Earth, Sun, stars, galaxies, but not with the entire Universe. Each object can pick up the energy and elevate the mortal life to immortal level, and keep it for a while. Immortality is not a name of the process, but the stage of the personal energy.

Do not look on mortal people as on the obsolete form of human being. You are on the age with mortals, and can become mortal any time, when you lose the track of your personal energy.

It is the universal law that is the same everywhere. Mortal people, and any mortal objects don't bother to manage the personal energy, and die sooner or later, becoming the parts of other mortal or immortal objects. The beauty of immortal life is the knowledge about the universal law, and ability to elevate life up to the highest level possible.

Therefore, our Universe is such a beautiful, and immortal. Go up in every moment, and never come lower, being honorable part of immortal world.

After connecting with Allen, I always feel my energy becomes higher. Why I asked him such a question, being in dissonance with myself? He didn't tell me anything, that I didn't know, but I was on lower energy level, and lost my vision for a moment. Allen restored my energy and vision over the network.

Same things happen, when I help other immortals to gain energy back over the network.

The outcome could be, that mortal world is very close to us, and represents the entropy of the world. Immortal life is not a gift of the nature, but the obligation of every human to resist the entropy with the full range of available knowledge.

What would be more attractive, that beautiful life that newer ends? It is a dream of any-one, but who going to believe, that this dream can become true?

My friends told me, that good things do newer last long, and can be easily spoiled by jealous people. Immortal life cannot be spoiled by anyone due to the idea of immortality. Immortal people, who believe in it, are not jealous, and mortal people, who could be jealous, do not believe in immortal life.

Immortality is an object and method of research. Each new step brings the questions, and new body calls. Objects by itself become the matter of investigation, and not the illusory curtains that we hang on the objects.

Who could know us better than we, ourselves? No one can bring the wisdom of immortality to us, except us. The network, that is uniting us, is the collective consciousness that becomes accessible only for immortals to promote the collective personal energy.

What would be our future? Immortals don't think about future, since we are enjoying the immortal life today, now, in the same moment we live. Why we need to care about the future? The future is the mortal concern, since only mortals expecting better future, than the past, or presence. The future is created today, and will be as bright as it is now.

How far can go the human's evolution? Would be the immortals different, and not the same, as mortal people?

Immortals are already different in many aspects. I see them, and they see me changing each day for better. Are any limitations for changes?

Probably, not. The Universe exists in very different conditions. Humans were born in special conditions on the Earth, and, possibly, will go far beyond these conditions to approach to the Universe variety.

It could happen sooner or later, and we will travel much farther away from the place, where we were born, if we would need it.

Immortal objects accelerate the natural selection in the Universe, and promote life even faster than it is now.

Life in Universe accelerates itself with speed much higher than speed of light. The complexity of Universal energy jumps like an explosion, and we are the part of this explosion. This process is endless, and it is as it was long time ago. Immortals are ever existing objects, as it was long time ago, and as it is now. The immortal network is also endless, and ever existing in our immortal life. We can connect to Universe by getting the adequate energy for it.

Growing population of immortal people here, on Earth, is the part of the accelerated natural selection. This process exists on the Earth along the millions of years, and immortals mutate to accommodate the new environment.

Can immortals reject the mortal world, as the lower form of life? It would be a mistake to ignore the mortal world that is the source of the immortal world. Universe can't reject part of itself, since it is senseless.

Journey in Darkness

My lovely son died in the age of twenty-eight, leaving us with unbearable pain of loss and grief. It was the test of my immortal energy that supposed to protect me from getting illness or becoming crazy.

By the going to the upper age of my suffering mind, I understand, that all heaviness of my emotional hurricane is not going deep in my body and stays on the surface of my energy in form of cry and tears.

The impact on my immortal life was huge and can't be managed by my mind and will. All my personality was paralyzed, and I wish only one – make my son be alive again. My immortal energy was not enough to make my son alive, and I feel, that I completely failed as immortal person, who wasn't able to promote life in my own family.

What was my excuse? I offered my help to son, and he rejected it, because I offered none traditional way to cure his disease. He believes only in conventional medical treatment that failed to help him. Mortal people are living in darkness of disbelieve, and hoping to get help from empty sources. It was the case, where I was not able to pass my knowledge to my own son. Hundred times I feel guilt that I can't find proper approach to his mind to give him my inspiration. It was too late to look for excuses, and my heart was squeezed by the grief and sorrow.

Immortal life is like a germinated seed that gives a new bright green leaf on the burned ground of grief. My energy restores itself in short term that was negatively accepted by my family, accusing me in not sufficient love to my son. I love him more than my life, but my life can't be cancelled in any way, being eternal. What could I do?

I feel like I am carrying my son inside of me and giving him his new life through my power. Wat it was? My madness, or call of my eternity, I can't explain it.

My family was so much depressed that were afraid even go on cemetery and see the grave of our son. I was alone staying on the age of freshly closed burial place with flowers in my hand and pulsing blood in my head. I feel, that I must be close to son's grave, as soon as possible, by hearing his thin voice coming to me from the above. My understanding of human's soul is very limited, and I didn't believe in it. The voice of my son was so much real and persistent, that I can't resist to go and be close to him.

Something happened after I came back home. I was agitated, nervous, and can't concentrate.

On the next day, I feel and see him inside of me. I drive my car to the parking lot and almost couldn't see anything, except the face of my son. At work I see him constantly and trying to switch my attention on my day to day duties. He shows me something by his hands by rising and lowering his palms. His face was smiling, and his ayes express the willingness to tell me important thing.

I was so sad and happy to see him that was not able to understand his body language. Later, at home, I carefully talked to my wife about my vision, being afraid that she will decide that I got completely crazy.

She watched my movements, and explain me, that my son asked us to be safe and don't warry about him.

Later I see my son inside of me without attempts to tell me anything, but rather thinking about some important things, that I don't know.

Time, yoga, and meditations, moves me and my family from the horror of life to the new life.

The Universe don't wish us to die, and the Journey to darkness comes to the end.

Recovery

Our children are connected to us more than anything in the world and losing them causes severe damage in the personal energy. How to restore something that was permanently gone from our life?

Grief, as the most acute form of emotional pain, cures our souls by itself. Extreme pain makes our brain blind to prevent its damage. Day by day our energy recovers itself and we start to understand what happens, and why we are in such pain.

Some mortals are not able to accept the pain, and taking pain killers, or psychotic medications, depends on the source of pain. I found, that getting medications tranquilize people, but not resolve the source of grief.

Only getting new energy from the different sources can restore such a significant energy loss as losing child. Nothing can bring child back, but the hole in the personal energy can be gradually filled by the multiple other sources of energy existing in the Universe.

I see my child in other people and let my sympathy to bring it closer to me. I see sun, grass, birds in the sky, and listen to natural sounds that symbolize life and cure me from the grief. I feel that my son is everywhere, in each molecule of the things surrounding me, and I love this world even stronger than before.

Nothing happens without purpose in this world. We must be attentive to the will of life and think about beauty and love.

I can't think about anything else, except the love to my son and the entire Universe that exists now and will exist ever.

My eternity brings me much higher up. I can't expect such fast grows of my personal energy from my exercises. Extreme pain makes me a different person and opens a new vision on my life.

Each way is different, we are going to live longer, and bring our love to the entire world. You are getting back what was lost in the past.

Sun and love are for everyone.

Bitterness and Unhappiness

Two dangerous symptoms: bitterness and constant unhappiness can destroy person's life. Be attentive to people who are constantly unhappy, none satisfy, often complaining, and looking for different way to be satisfied. These two symptoms of low energy are also accompanied by anger and fear.

People with a set of such symptoms are dangerously ill and could be drug addicted. Drugs stimulate the excretion of hormones that are missing in the blood, and make person a bit happier for short period of time. People become "softer" and "warmer" in feelings and relations with the other people. Using drugs makes the illness even worse.

How to help these straggling people to elevate the positive mood, and stand away from toxic drugs?

The following recommendations good for mortal people since immortals are not the subject of bad mood illnesses.

The breathing yoga exercises are good for accumulation energy in the entire body. Physical yoga distributes the accumulated energy in mind and body making it more susceptible for feeling of happiness. Meditation helps to escape bad mental considerations about "senseless life".

Performing Energy Circle extends the personal energy to the level where illness have gone, and positive acceptance of life is dominating.

Your intention to fight the "low mood" illness will end up with success, and you will see the beauty of life everywhere.

Isolation and Loneliness

Lack of personal energy can be experienced as isolation and loneliness. Nothing could satisfy you, if your energy is low. People try to satisfy themselves by buying different expensive things, including cars, properties, jewelries, food, clothe, etc. It doesn't work since the reason of loneliness is not in the insufficient amount of "positive" stimulus, but in the missing connection with the Universal Energy.

Mortal people often surround themselves with the excess of different objects that supposed to create positive influence on the mood. As a result, it is only objects of your life, and it is not the sources of the universal energy. To get connected to the real source of joy, you need to meditate on the vibration of the universal energy that melts the ice of loneliness and isolation.

Your friends, relatives, parents, and all what you love in this world would not help you to recover from the darkness of isolation, if you will not resonate with the energy of the people and love them with all your heart. Isolation and loneliness are not the situation in your life, when everyone is turning away from you, but the loss of connection with energy of people who loves you and are ready to help. Hugging does not necessarily means loving. Love is the main remedy against the isolation and loneliness. Love is the result of resonance with the energy of other objects, including people, plants, animals, Earth, and the entire world.

Mortal people could be lonely in the crowd of people being detached from them. People with insufficient energy can reject love of people who loves them. Loneliness is the serious symptom of insufficient energy that must be cured as soon as possible.

You should start to perform energy exercises if you feel like you are living in the pipe of isolation.

Immortals newer experiencing isolation or loneliness being in touch with the entire world, and even prefer to be alone to reduce the excess of interaction with other people.

Immortal Life Against the Euthanasia and Suicide

Why so many people taking they life voluntarily? Is life of some people appearing to be so bad that they wish to end it by themselves or by someone's help?

Yes, it is the fact that we can't ignore. People don't want to live due to number of reasons, and one of it is suffer of physical or emotional pain. Unbearable pain exhausts the human being and makes him the prisoner of circumstances.

Pain in body or in soul symbolizes destruction and illness that should be cured by applying certain procedures. Medical procedure usually considered the first aid by pain, but elevation the personal energy is the powerful alternative way for pain reduction.

Pain means the body call to cure. Artificial reduction of pain, in any way, means ignorance of giving cure to person. It is the same as the emergency operator is hanging up on you when you making emergency call for help.

Regular pain reduction leads to fatal end, when person experience such enormous pain that is not able to manage it anymore asking for death as one possible escape from it.

Can immortals help in this case? For all people, who suffer from physical or emotional pain, the way to escape the crucial stage always exists. Never stop your life in any circumstances, in any good or bad mood, by suggestions of anyone, or experiencing strong physical pain, or suffering from psychological pain, shame and disbelieve. All of it is your imagination, temporary blindness, and personal energy loss. It is always fixable by performing simple procedures, where you open your contracted energy centers to such powerful source of energy as the Universe.

Perform yoga breath, vipassana meditation, and Energy Circle to restore your energy immediately and get some relief on the spot. Practice these simple exercises as many times as you can, enter your pain, facilitate it, and let it work for you. Ask yourself about your fears and coldness. Look for the source of your discomfort and anxiety by asking deeper and deeper questions until you reach the core of problem. Direct your personal energy on it, as you aim the flashlight on dark place. Use professional help of people, who can assess your pain and warries to find proper healing by improving your personal energy.

Life is a gift of god, and god can cure you when you open your face to him. The Universal energy makes any type of death unreasonable and unethical. Join the Immortal Society instead of "dying with dignity...", since any type of death cannot be associated with dignity, where only life can be respectful.

What Happens with Mortal People After Death?

This question has always interested me, and I was the one who supported the Omton's idea about the entire disintegration of person and the personal energy after the death. It constitutes the uselessness of mortal life and adds tragedy of the human's death.

I was always referring to my mental model of a mortal person who died, and try to explain my vision of the dead as the vision of existing person. Omton explains it as an activation of my memory that assembles the image in my mind since nothing has been remained after the death.

My son passed away in the time when my personal energy was on the rise and gives me the moments of vision that I can't classify as something that I could create in my imagination. It was absolute real contact with my son, similar that I experience when I am contacting living immortals over the network. He was contacting me as alive person. I was shocked by the reality of the communication, and call Allen to discuss this case.

Allen was quietly sitting in my room without showing any emotions, and I feel very relaxing in his presence. He was meditating on my statement about afterlife people' activity. I closed my eyes and waited for his response.

After the time I opened my eyes and see Allen smilingly observing my face.

"Did you get some energy?" – asked he.

I confirmed it and asked him to proceed with his opinion on my observations.

Allen was in complicated situation, because he, certainly, didn't believe in afterlife, but he trusted my feelings, and wish to support me in this difficult for me time. I know that Allen will newer give me the false statement only to calm me down or satisfy my expectations.

Finally, he told me that I was right about my feelings, and people are not losing personal energy immediately after the death but continue to be interacting with the world using the remedy that is unknown to us. They can feel, see, and experience the world in the way that is like what we can experience being alive.

I was barely shocked by Allen's words and feel enormous relief in my soul. Allen confirmed that he was wrong about complete person's destruction following the death and asked me to assist him in getting knowledge about my experience with contacting my son. He also mentioned that similar cases have been reported to him by other immortals and this all cannot be someone's imagination, but rather real experience of something that is outside of our understanding of what is life and death.

I was able to contact my son after several months of his death. Sometimes I try to initiate a contact by meditating on his energy being an initiator of the contact. Often, I feel his presence and desire to contact me in form of merging my personal energy to his energy. The second form of contact was much more effective in terms of vision of his presence.

First time I found him in dark and wet tunnel. He was disoriented and confused trying to contact me in any way. His eyes were not able to see me, and he didn't talk to me. None regards with it, he was recognized my presence and turned his face towards me.

I was devastated by seeing him in such condition and take his hands in my palms to let him follow to the light in the far end of the tunnel. He certainly didn't see the light and can't understand where he is. I let him step towards me and slowly approach the exit from tunnel.

Next time I found my son in the same condition, and in the same place. I approached to him again and take his palms in my palms to move further. We continue to move several days until the tunnel comes to the end. The place outside tunnel was gray and I see bright light coming from the horizon like from the sun.

After several days we continue to move towards the light and the gray fog, surrounded us, gradually disappeared. I see the seclude piece of land, covered by sand and stones. The light becomes very bright and hot. It stops me from moving any further since I see sparks emanated from my son's astral body. I was afraid to lose him being dissolved in this bright light.

Next time I found my son sitting in meditation in the same place under very bright light. I approached to him, and he raised. We start to move ahead, and see the valley covered by fog. The road starts to go down in the foggy space with dark branches of dead trees hidden in the fog.

The patches of fog become more translucent closer to the valley bottom, and we approached to the wooden house staying beside the road. Some people dressed in clothe of 18th century was sitting around the table on the patio and silently watching us.

We stopped our movement and returned to the original place. The foggy valley appeared for us scary and unpleasant. I left my son in the same place where I found him in this time.

After several hours I try to contact him again to move him further, but he refuses and continue to sit in the same pose. The time is going, but he didn't move any further, and it disturbs me a little. He sent me a message that time in his world is going differently compare with my world. He is not in rush to make his own decision and ignores my attempts to accelerate his new life.

What pushes us to live faster? We always try to be on time, do not miss the opportunity, and suffer from time loss. Why is that? What happens if we will not accelerate the life? Who will come first to the finish? Who wins the price? What is the price that we are straggling to win?

Many questions were raised in my head after conversation with my son. I tried to accelerate his life when he lived in my world by giving him some "good" advises, that I consider being "good", because it will accelerate his life. For what?

Now I lost him and my "acceleration" comes to the dust. Does my own acceleration become a dust at the certain time?

As an immortal person, I am living in the resonance with the energy of the universe that is not related to the pace of my life. I am happy no matter how strong I push my life ahead since I am doing it in meditation that is above any "acceleration".

Rush in life is the result of living with blindness. We are jumping back and forward in our mind to find the "better" solution, but it is already in our mind, and we don't see it. Meditation stops our mental craziness and reveals the truth.

Million times I asked what happened with my son when I lost him, and my mind collapsed in attempts to understand the reality straggling in pain and grief. Meditation brings me the clear vision of what happens, and pacified my mind. Everyone has natural rights to live in the space where one likes to live, and where god places us when time is coming. We cannot negotiate with god about better future or past. We can love god, and be in joyful light of love, but we can't guarantee this joy to anyone who depends on us since the "dependency" is a miracle. Each soul, or personal energy, grows by itself being in resonance with god and entire world. Can we share our energy with anyone? Possibly not, but we can share our experience with other people to let them know that the joy of love really exists and cures all difficulties in our life.

Grief is blind and serves our ego in feeling of loss. At the certain point in struggle, being in meditation, I understand that only my ego misses my son who left our world. He was chosen by god to go in different place to continue his ascending being in astral energy. Why I should be against it? It happens occasionally, and I wasn't being prepared to it, but I should respect the god's will and appreciate the reality. Immortal people must understand the beauty of real world that looks as ugly place to others.

Day after, I visited my son again and found him sitting in the same place on bright light. He becomes more cooperative in this time and raises his hand in greeting. I take his hand in my, and he raised being ready to follow me. We move ahead in the desert towards the light. The valley with foggy trees was left aside the road. The light becomes even brighter by our movement, and I see the small sparks coming from our bodies. These sparks fly around us as the shiny insects and rotate making the shape of sphere. The surrounding has been changed and I found small vegetation growing between the stones. We walked several miles together, and then stop in the same place where we started to move without any idea where to go. I feel myself disoriented and helpless before to lose the contact.

Several days in a row I was not be able to restore meaningful contact with my son. I see him sitting in the same place without paying attention on my presence. I try to rise him to walk together, but he didn't raise, and continue sitting.

I was thinking that he probably is going in the same stage as me. We both are in the first stage of immortal life. His time is going not as fast as the time in my space, but we both are meditating on the personal energy.

Who pushes me to move towards the eternity? I don't know, and he, probably, doesn't know by himself. Most certainly that it is the natural process of personal proliferation that walks us from darkness of unknown to the light of knowledge. We are getting knowledge from meditation and move ahead being in stage of eureka.

My son becomes more advanced than me being in the stage of pure meditation. I was straggle in pain of loss and attachment to the things in my life being unable to free myself from predetermined love to some objects.

I feel how weak becomes my personal energy and my body becomes heavy and rigid. My regular smile comes out of my face, and I see myself in dark cloud of uncertainty. How to regain my previous life when I was in good progress in immortal living? Why god picked me for this harsh test? Why other members of my family should share my grief and suffer? What is it all for?

I learned that nothing happens in my life without reason, and some reason must be in my son's death. Does god kill, to save? If yes, then who was saved? We will never understand it since our vision is narrow due to the limited time of observation. I try to improve my vision to see the things that happen in my life, but there is a lot of uncertainty anyway.

Every day I visit my son and try to help him to gain a new form of life. Does he need me on his way? Probably yes, since he contacted me strongly in the beginning. His attachment to me becomes weaker over the time, and I see that he can manage his life by himself denying my involvement. The surrounding environment changes each time becoming softer and more pleasant. He was surrounded by fresh vegetation growing between stones, and the space was saturated by tiny gray particles that reduce the brightness of light.

The changes, that I was witnessed, conclude the independence of the personal life from the universal life that unites us in one living world. Why we need to be born and die later to continue our life in the other world? Why this circle is running in the universe?

Circle of Life

I could consider the contact with my son as the form of my imagination that helps me to cure my grief and exist only in my brain. Allen didn't explain his vision of afterlife existence, but rather walk away from this theme.

Today Allen visited me and let me know his theory of afterlife. He accounted my emotional status and talked to me in soft and respectful way to prevent possible misunderstanding.

How could anyone live after the death? What would be such life looks like? Can people feel anything or use the brain for intellectual activity? Many questions must be answered and there is no way to confirm or reject the truth since no one can contact the afterlife being in conscious state.

Allen stayed quietly several minutes, and then continued his explanation. He confirms my ability to see my son and helping him to progress in the other world, but only in my brain that creates my son's image in form of personal energy that creates vibrations, restores and amplifies vibrations in the universe by creating image of my son. This is the way that my son continues to live. I am the generator of my son's afterlife, but nothing more. My wife creates her image of our son that is not the same as mine image that proves the Allen's theory.

"You create the most possible image of your lovely one that explains your understanding of the afterlife, and therefore your son can't see you there or talk to you there. You alone create his environment in the way as you wish. This is the real afterlife that truly exists." – Concluded Allen.

I was sad to know that all my action was my illusion, and only my imagination. Allen takes my hand and his eyes look deeply in my eyes going inside in my brain and helping me to restore my energy.

"You and your wife gave him life once, and now you are giving it again" – told Allen.

My son is alive in another world as long as I help him to be alive. It means that nothing really exists after person's death, only memory in mind of people who love, or simply know the person.

"What do you think is your memory?" – asked Allen.

"More or less stable links in my brain" – was my answer.

"What are these links for?" – He asked again.

"To memorize objects and events, I guess".

"Are these objects and events real?"

"No, it is only my imagination."

"Can you imagine that you newer had your son?"

"No, I can't."

"It means that your imagination doesn't belong to your will."

"Why? My imagination is only my fantasy, and nothing else."

"Your imagination is the reflection of the reality, and nothing else. You create the reality and live in it in the same way as you live in your room. There is no difference in your perception and understanding. Your reality becomes independent from your imagination and you just participate in it without any fantasy. Your son is very much alive and communicates with you as the real person. It is not the "fantasy", you cannot change your vision by your will."

I stay silent trying to digest Allen's words. The sweet feeling of my son's presence captured my mind and I smiled in my dreams about him.

"What if I die? Would my son still alive in other world?" – asked I.

"He will, being recalled by some-one's mind that will produce vibrations making him alive again. – I hope that you will never die." – add Allen.

"Allen, does he feel anything when I am contacting him?"

"Yes, he feels in the same way as you and me, and we see it by contacting him."

"Why he becomes more independent from me by the time is passed?" – asked I.

"It is you, who becomes more independent from him, and need his attention only when contact is established." – was his answer.

"How long he will be contacting me?"

"You will be with him forever."

Allen raised from his chare and makes several steps towards me.

"You will live with son as long as your life will be in progress, and newer stop see him in his journey to perfection. Do not miss him but be happy for him who is in constant progress now."

Allen left, and, in my mind, I see him taking an elevator on my floor, elevator's door had been opened and my wife stepped out the cabin. They greeted each other, and door was closed. I realized that my wife is dressed in her beautiful dress with green flowers on it that she liked to wear in the past but now placed deeply in the closed after our son's death. Immediately I hear the ring in my door entrance and raised from the chair to open the door. I see my wife wearing her beautiful dress with green flowers. I hugged her and whispered several times "He is alive … He is alive".

I know since then that our son is alive and waiting for our contact. He is so far away, and he is so close to us as he was never before.

Serge Dobrow

References

1. Allen Omton "The Theory and Practice of Immortality". Amazon. 2017.
2. Allen Omton "Start Your Eternal Life". Amazon. 2018.